7 Days to Get Back to Sleep

Summary

Who am I?

My name is Jonathan White and I wrote this mini guide, because I am a specialist in sleep medicine. I have helped thousands of people get back to sleep by applying simple and practical methods and techniques.

I realized that unfortunately, many people were struggling with insomnia and finding a lasting solution to their problem was difficult for them. So, I decided to write this mini guide to help them get back to sleep in 7 days.

I have leveraged my expertise and experience to develop this powerful and accessible program. This guide contains exercises and practical advice for getting to know yourself better and optimizing your lifestyle in order to sleep better. I hope it will help readers to naturally and long-term regain their sleep.

Good reading!
Jonathan.

DISCLAIMER

The content of this mini-guide is provided for informational purposes only and should not be considered as a diagnosis or treatment for any form of insomnia. The information contained in this mini-guide should under no circumstances replace a medical opinion.

If you are suffering from insomnia, please consult a qualified professional to determine the cause, severity, and appropriate treatment. The information provided in this mini-guide is based on the author's personal experience and knowledge, but does not necessarily represent general guidelines for all cases of insomnia.

We do not guarantee that the strategies and methods suggested will work for you and cannot be held responsible if these strategies and methods do not produce the desired results.

Day 1: Define the Problem

On the first day of your journey to better sleep, you start by defining the problem. What is causing your insomnia? Are you having difficulty falling asleep or difficulty staying asleep? Or maybe both? Is this an issue that has been around for a while or is it new?

When trying to understand what's causing your insomnia, you should look into the stressors and environmental factors that may be affecting your nights.

Some stress factors can include:

- A Bad Day at Work

- Relationship Issues

- Financial Difficulties

- Health Issues

- Concern about uncertain situations

- Overtaxing oneself, having an irregular schedule, and frequent changes to routines can also be sources of stress.

- Regarding environmental factors, you should analyze the room. Your bedroom should be a sanctuary. Your bed should be a place where you can relax and where you can sleep without being disturbed by external factors such as noise, light, odors, temperature, and humidity.

You should also examine your bedtime routines. Check what you're doing each night before bed and if it has an impact on your sleep. Should you make changes to these habits to help you sleep better?

You should also examine your diet and caffeine consumption. Avoid drinking coffee or caffeinated drinks after 4 pm. Additionally, try to eat healthily and balanced and avoid consuming high-fat foods before bed.

Finally, it is important to consider physical activity. Regular physical activity can help to improve the quality of sleep and prevent insomnia. However, make sure not to do exercises too close to bedtime as this can prevent you from falling asleep.

Thus, in order to understand what is causing your insomnia, you will need to examine sources of stress, environmental factors, and your bedtime habits. Once you have understood what is causing your insomnia, you can begin to find solutions to help you sleep better and put an end to the insomnia.

Understanding the Causes of Insomnia

Understanding the causes of insomnia can help find solutions to regain restorative and lasting sleep. Insomnia, which is often part of a set of sleep disorders, can have several different causes.

The main causes of insomnia are as follows:

- Mental and emotional distress: disorders such as depression and anxiety can lead to difficulty falling asleep or maintaining sleep.

- Environmental factors: noise and light can influence the quality and duration of sleep.

- Medication: Some medications can cause sleep disorders.

- Bad sleeping habits: sleeping at irregular hours or sleeping for too long can lead to difficulty in falling asleep and staying asleep.

- Eating Habits: Foods consumed at the wrong times or products containing caffeine can interfere with sleep.

- Chronic illnesses: some illnesses such as sleep apnea or fibromyalgia can cause sleep disorders.

- Sleep-wake rhythm disorders: For people suffering from sleep-wake rhythm disorders, sleep can be very disrupted.

- Age: Sleep can be affected by aging and age-related changes.

- Personal and professional issues: Personal or professional problems can interfere with sleep.

In conclusion, understanding the causes of insomnia is essential in order to find solutions to regain restorative and lasting sleep. By identifying and treating underlying causes, it is possible to improve the quality of sleep and overall well-being.

Understanding the Sleep Cycle

Sleep is a complex process essential for health and quality of life. It is a cycle of phases that follow each other during the night. Learning to understand the sleep cycle is the first step to be able to master it and regain optimal sleep.

The Stages of the Sleep Cycle

The sleep cycle consists of two main phases: the wake phase and the deep sleep phase. The wake phase is the stage where the person is awake and conscious, while the deep sleep phase is the stage where the brain is less active and the body is completely relaxed. In between these two phases, there are four other stages of sleep:

- Light sleep stage: This stage is characterized by a slower heart and respiratory rate and a decrease in muscle activity.

- Stage 3: This is the stage where deep sleep begins to manifest. It is characterized by greater relaxation and the onset of dreaming.

- Stage 4: This stage is the deepest stage of sleep and is characterized by very low brain activity.

- Stage 5: This stage is the stage of paradoxical sleep and is characterized by a very high level of brain activity and very rapid eye movements.

Duration of Sleep Cycle

The sleep cycle lasts approximately 90 minutes. Each cycle is composed of several stages and each stage lasts about 20 minutes. During one night, a person can go through five to six sleep cycles. It is therefore important to understand the sleep cycle in order to plan adequate sleep hours and have good quality of sleep.

Benefits of Sleep

Sleep is very important for the body and mind. It allows the body to regenerate and heal. It also allows the mind to rest and function properly. A good night's sleep helps to improve concentration and memory, reduce stress and enhance physical and mental performance.

Daily Habits

In order to understand the sleep cycle, it is important to take into account daily habits. It is important to maintain a sleep routine, going to bed and getting up at the same time each day. It is also important to limit the consumption of caffeine and other stimulants, as well as the consumption of alcohol and other substances that can interfere with the sleep cycle. Furthermore, it is important to practice regular physical activity and to adopt relaxation techniques to relax and facilitate falling asleep.

Finally, it is important to create a conducive environment for restorative sleep: a dark, cool and quiet room and a comfortable mattress and pillows. Maintaining a sleep routine and eating a healthy and balanced diet is also essential to ensure that the sleep cycle is optimal.

Understanding the Negative Effects of Insomnia

Insomnia is a sleep disorder affecting many people and can have detrimental effects on health. It is often associated with significant consequences on the quality of life of those affected, both emotionally and physically, as well as socially and professionally.

To start, it is important to understand that insomnia is a symptom and not a disease in itself. Insomnia is usually linked to other factors such as stress, anxiety, physical or mental health issues, taking certain medications, lifestyle changes, and other factors.

Due to the harmful effects of insomnia, it is important to take the necessary measures to understand its causes and adopt methods to remedy it. Here are a few:

- Increase the levels of serotonin and dopamine in your body. These two chemicals are involved in mood and sleep regulation.
- Adapt your environment to your sleep. This means improving your bedroom to make it more conducive to your sleep, such as having a suitable temperature, a suitable paint color, a comfortable mattress, minimal lighting, soothing sounds, etc.
- Change your diet. Eating foods that promote sleep can greatly help improve your sleep. This includes foods high in tryptophan, vitamin B6, magnesium, and zinc.
- Reducing Stress. Stress management can have a big impact on your sleep. Try practicing relaxation exercises or relaxation methods such as meditation and deep breathing.
- Practicing physical activity. Moderate physical activity can help to relieve stress and improve the quality of your sleep.
- Limit the use of media and electronic devices. The blue lights from televisions, computers, and phones stimulate the brain and can disrupt your sleep.

Finally, it is also important to consult a doctor if you are suffering from insomnia. They can help you understand the causes of your insomnia and develop a treatment plan tailored to your situation.

Day 2: Habits to Take On

The second day is dedicated to habits to take to be able to end insomnia and get back to sleep. In this new stage of the program, we will put in place rituals and habits that will allow you to sleep better and feel more rested.

First of all, it is important not to oversleep during the day. Although sleeping is beneficial, daytime sleepiness can have negative effects on night-time sleep. So avoid taking naps and if you feel yourself getting sleepy, get up and do an activity that keeps you awake.

Likewise, avoid taking drinks containing caffeine. Caffeine can have a negative impact on sleep as it is a stimulant that causes a reduction in sleep quality.

Finally, try to get up and go to bed at regular hours. Developing a sleep routine can help you fall asleep more easily and wake up more rested. In this routine, try to avoid activities that can excite you, such as watching movies or series or playing video games.

In order to prepare yourself for a better night's sleep, it is also helpful to develop relaxing rituals. For example, you can lie down and do a session of deep breathing, do some light physical activity, read a book, or listen to some calming music. These activities will help you to relax and better prepare yourself for sleep.

Finally, before going to bed, try to disconnect from screens. Screens, especially computers and cell phones, are usually sources of stimulation that can interfere with your sleep. It is therefore advisable to stay away from screens at least an hour before going to bed.

By following these few tips, you can prepare yourself for deeper and more restorative sleep.

Establish a Sleep Schedule

The sleep rhythm is essential for getting a good quality of sleep. It is therefore vital to create a regular sleep schedule, a bedtime and wake-up routine that suits your body.

In order to create a sleep rhythm that suits your body, you must:

- Establish a regular sleep schedule: set a consistent bedtime and wake-up time even on weekends. Try to go to bed and wake up at the same time every day.

- Go to bed only when you're tired: don't force yourself to sleep, you might wake up earlier in the morning. If you can't fall asleep, try to relax by reading a book, listening to music or taking a warm bath.

- Use an alarm clock rather than relying on restorative sleep: when you fall into the arms of Morpheus, it's harder to regulate the time at which you wake up, so plan your sleep and set your alarm.

- Avoid taking too long naps: naps can be very beneficial but be careful not to oversleep; it can affect your sleep quality at night.

- Avoid substances that disrupt sleep: alcohol, tobacco, and certain medications can have negative effects on your sleep. Limit stimulants, such as caffeine, early in the day.

- Avoid stimulating activities before bedtime: video games, physical and intellectual tasks such as crosswords, and stress can be stimulating and prevent you from falling asleep.

- Create a peaceful environment: your bedroom should be quiet, dark, and cool. Use curtains and blinds to block out light, a humidifier to maintain humidity, and candles if necessary.

- Exercising regularly: Exercise can help you feel more tired in the evening and sleep better at night. Choose non-stimulating activities such as walking, swimming, yoga or stretching, and try to do them early in the morning or in the late afternoon.

- Prepare a hot drink before going to bed: chamomile, mint tea or warm milk can help you relax and make it easier to fall asleep.

- Limit the use of electronic devices before bedtime: the blue lights of screens can be very stimulating and affect the quality of your sleep. Try to turn off all electronic devices an hour before going to bed.

By taking these precautions, you can create an adequate sleep rhythm and feel more rested and ready to face the day.

Relaxation Techniques

Today, we will discuss relaxation techniques which are essential to getting a good night's sleep. It is essential to take a break and find ways to calm both the body and mind to get the sleep you need.

Relaxation techniques can vary greatly, but they all have the same goal - to develop a serene and peaceful awareness that encourages relaxation and sleep. Here are some examples of relaxation techniques to try:

- Meditation: Meditation is an effective form of relaxation that seeks to clear your mind of any thoughts and distractions that might keep you from sleeping. It is recommended to meditate for about 10 to 15 minutes before bed to relax.

- Deep Breathing: This technique helps to release muscle tension and relieve stress. Slowly and deeply breathe for five minutes, being aware of each of your breaths.

- Yoga: Yoga has many benefits for your health. In addition to helping you relax and unwind, it helps you to breathe better and manage stress. It is recommended to practice yoga before going to bed to enjoy its benefits.

- Massage: Massages are great for getting rid of tensions and muscular pain which might prevent sleep. You can massage yourself or ask a partner to massage you.

- Positive Imaginations: It can be helpful to recall pleasant, happy moments to relax tension and let the mind settle. Let your mind wander and imagine yourself in a pleasant situation that helps you sleep better.

- Relaxing Music: Listening to relaxing music can help to calm your mind and relax more easily. You can choose calm and melodious pieces to help you relax and sleep better.

- Hot Baths and Other Methods: A hot bath or a hot shower can help ease tension and relax muscles. You can also try heat wraps or hot foot baths to help you relax.

Finally, don't forget that you can also try visualization exercises to help you relax. Visualize yourself sailing in a vast ocean or in a lush forest. This can help you channel your energy and better relax.

In conclusion, relaxation techniques are essential for regaining sleep. It is important to find ways to relax your body and mind to help you sleep better and feel better. Try different methods to find the one that suits you best and will help you have a better sleep.

Avoid Stimulants

To get back to sleep and put an end to insomnia, it is essential to stay away from stimulants. Stimulants can be consumed through drinks or food products, but also environmental. Stimulants can hinder our efforts to get back to sleep and interfere with our ability to fall asleep.

Here are some tips to avoid stimulants and get back to sleep:

- Avoid caffeine and tobacco. Caffeine can affect our ability to fall asleep and stay asleep. Caffeine is found in coffee, tea, soft drinks, and some energy drinks, and accumulates in our bodies for several hours, preventing us from falling asleep. Tobacco is also a stimulant and can affect our sleep by preventing us from falling asleep and staying asleep.
- Limit alcohol and physical activity before bedtime. Avoid alcohol as it can interfere with the quality of sleep. It can also have euphoric effects and hinder our ability to fall asleep. Likewise, intense physical activity just before bedtime can keep us awake and exhaust us.
- Limit exposure to light and screens before bedtime. Light can interfere with our internal clock and prevent us from falling asleep. Therefore, avoid exposure to blue light from screens such as televisions, phones, and computers before bedtime.

- Avoid foods high in sugar and fat before bedtime. Foods high in sugar and fat can interfere with our sleep and keep us awake. So avoid eating foods high in sugar and fat before bedtime.
- Try warm drinks and herbs. Warm drinks like hot milk or chamomile tea can help us relax and fall asleep. Also try herbs like valerian, lemon balm or lime tree which can help us to relax and fall asleep.
- Avoid taking naps and late night snacks. Naps can keep us awake and prevent us from falling asleep later at night. So, avoid taking naps and late night snacks to make it easier to fall asleep.
- Try relaxation exercises and deep breathing techniques. Try relaxation exercises and deep breathing techniques to help us relax and fall asleep. Short meditation sessions can also help us relax and get back to sleep.

By following these tips, it is possible to stay away from stimulants and regain sleep and put an end to insomnia.

Eat healthily and balanced

Eating healthy and balanced is an important part of the process to regain restorative and natural sleep. The foods that are consumed can have profound effects on the quality of sleep and how we feel it. It is essential to know what foods are good for sleep and what are the best eating habits to regain good sleep.

Start by adopting a healthy and varied diet, rich in fresh fruits and vegetables, whole grains, nuts, dairy products, lean meats, fish and healthy oils. These foods all contain the nutrients and vitamins your body needs to regenerate and recover. By limiting or avoiding processed foods, sugary drinks, fried foods and dairy products, you will feel more in tune with your body and your sleep.

Find nutrient-rich foods that contain essential vitamins and minerals for sleep, such as Vitamin B6, zinc, magnesium and iron. You can get these nutrients by eating foods such as bananas, nuts, chickpeas, fatty fish and leafy greens. Foods high in magnesium, zinc and Vitamin B6 can be useful for reducing anxiety and irritability and improving the quality of sleep.

Limit your consumption of protein-based products, as too much protein can lead to an increase in melatonin levels, which is the hormone that controls sleep. Also avoid consuming excessively sweet foods, which can cause a drop in your blood sugar levels and difficulty falling asleep.

Limit your caffeine intake as well, as it can stimulate the nervous system and cause sleep disturbances. Try not to consume caffeine after 5 PM and make sure to drink enough liquids throughout the day to stay hydrated and ease sleep.

Avoid eating heavily just before bedtime, as this can lead to disturbances in sleep. A light and healthy snack before bedtime can be safe and even beneficial for sleep. Dried fruits, dairy products, nuts and seeds are examples of healthy snacks that can be consumed close to bedtime.

Finally, try to eat at regular times and stick to your eating schedule. This can help regulate sleep cycles and improve the quality and length of sleep. Try to eat at fixed times and consume healthy and varied foods at each meal to promote good sleep.

Day 3: Practices to Adopt

On Day 3, you will begin to notice changes and results in your sleep. But this is not the time to slack off, you will have to keep applying certain practices to maintain these results.

Sleep is a process, not an action. Therefore, in order to get back to sleep, it is necessary to understand the basics of good health and good sleep habits.

Here are some practices to adopt:

- Create a peaceful and uninterrupted sleep environment. Use blackout curtains, earplugs, a humidifier, etc. to eliminate noise and lights that prevent restorative sleep.

- Avoid stimulants before going to bed. Avoid caffeine and alcohol in the evening and do not smoke before bedtime as this will stimulate your brain and body and prevent you from finding sleep.

- Develop a bedtime routine. Try to go to bed at the same time every night and avoid late naps.

- Do yoga or light movements before bed. This slows your heart rate and helps to promote calmness.

- Take a warm bath before bed. It can help to loosen up the muscles and reduce stress.

- Use a low-light lamp in your bedroom. This helps to signal to your body that it's time to sleep.

- Avoid using screens near your bed. Artificial light can interfere with your sleep.

- Listen to calming and relaxing music before going to bed. It will help to soothe your mind and help you fall asleep faster.

- Try relaxation techniques such as sleep yoga, meditation, and visualization to help you relax.

- Write down your thoughts and worries before bed. This will relieve your mind and help you fall asleep faster.

- Drink a glass of milk before going to bed. Milk contains proteins and carbohydrates that promote sleep.

- Try some deep breathing techniques to relax. This can help to soothe your body and mind.

- Don't be afraid to ask for help if you're still having trouble sleeping. It is possible to consult a sleep specialist to help you find personalized solutions.

It is essential to adopt these practices to regain healthy and restorative sleep. With time and perseverance, you will soon be able to regain your balance and enjoy a deep and restorative sleep.

Conscious Breathing:

Conscious breathing is a practice that allows access to inner calm and to regain restorative sleep. By becoming aware of your breath, you will learn to better relax your body and to release the stress and anxiety that can be the cause of your insomnia.

When you start practicing conscious breathing, begin by sitting or lying down in a comfortable position. Take a position in which you can feel at ease and relaxed, without too much tension in your body's muscles.

Breathe through your nose while being mindful of each inhalation and exhalation. Try to take deep breaths and fill your abdomen with oxygen. Feel the air entering your body and observe how your body responds to each breath. Focus on the air coming in and going out.

If your mind starts to wander, bring your attention back to your breath. Don't worry if you can't keep your focus for very long. Simply observe how your mind works.

You can also try to synchronize your breathing with your movement. Close your eyes and take a deep breath. Open your eyes and exhale. Repeat this exercise several times, trying to maintain a steady pace.

Conscious breathing can also be practiced during the day to release tension and find a state of calm and relaxation. For example, you can take a few minutes to take a break and enjoy this practice.

In conclusion, conscious breathing is a very simple practice and easy to incorporate into your daily routine. It can help you relax better and get a restorative sleep. So, take a few minutes every day to practice conscious breathing and reap the benefits it can have on your sleep.

Physical Exercise

Physical exercise is one of the most effective ways to help recover a restorative and healthy sleep. They are essential to stimulate melatonin, the sleep hormone, and to release the stress accumulated during the day. It is essential to train regularly to improve sleep and avoid insomnia.

Therefore, for the third day of this mini guide, we suggest for you to take advantage of the benefits of physical exercise to get back to sleep.

1. Practice cardiovascular exercises: a 30-minute session per day can stimulate the secretion of melatonin and release the stress hormone, cortisol. Cardiovascular activities include running, jogging, cycling, or skating.

2. Doing strength and conditioning activities: Strength and conditioning exercises can be very beneficial for getting to sleep faster and sleeping better. They also help

reduce stress and anxiety, and can be done two to three times a week.

3. Practice breathing and relaxation exercises: these exercises are very useful for calming the body and mind and relieving stress. One can learn a lot about yoga, meditation and mindfulness. It is recommended to practice these exercises for at least 10 to 15 minutes a day.

4. Do Zumba or Tai Chi: Zumba and Tai Chi are activities that provide a variety of benefits for the body and mind. It is important to choose classes suited to your level and goal, and to train at least two to three times a week.

5. Use apps to help you train: Training apps are an excellent solution for training at home or on the go. They can help you track your training and reach your health goals.

Finally, it is important to find a balance between exercise and rest. Listen to your body and respect your limits. Avoid training in the evening as it can affect your sleep. If you train in the evening, try to do it two hours before going to bed. Finally, take regular breaks to rest and relax.

Exposure to Daylight

Exposure to daylight is a fundamental element to get back to sleep. In fact, hours of exposure to light, and more precisely to daylight, are necessary to maintain a good biological rhythm.

To regulate your biological rhythm and take advantage of the benefits of daylight, here are a few steps to follow:

- Try to get up at a regular time, having a schedule that corresponds to your routine. By getting up at roughly the same time each day, your body will adjust to this new routine and you will have a better quality of sleep.

- Once you wake up, try to open the curtains and let the daylight in, which will be a signal for your body to adjust to this new schedule.

- Try to take your breakfast outside, or at least to go for a walk in a place full of light. This will help you feel more energized and for your biological rhythm to adapt to this new routine and schedule.

- If possible, try to have some physical activity outdoors, which will help boost your metabolism and biological rhythm, and help you have better quality sleep.

- Don't stay inside for too long, try to take a walk outside or go to a cafe or park to enjoy the sunlight.

- Avoid using the phone and screens before going to bed. The blue light emitted by these devices can disrupt your biological rhythm and make it difficult for you to fall asleep.

- Try to go to bed at a reasonable and consistent hour, and if possible in the dark. This will help you fall asleep more easily and have a better quality of sleep.

With these few tips, you should be able to get your sleep back and feel more rested and energized throughout the day. So, start enjoying the benefits of daylight and get the sleep you need.

Acupuncture and Yoga

Acupuncture and yoga are recognized practices for their relaxing effects and their ability to help restore restful sleep. To benefit from their effects, it is recommended to consult an acupuncturist doctor to guide you and assess the problem.

Acupuncture is a form of traditional Chinese medicine which involves the insertion of fine and secure needles at specific points of your body. The needles aim to create a flow within the body and to rebalance your energy to stimulate healing. Acupuncture can be very effective in relieving stress, muscle tension and anxiety associated with sleep disorders. It can also be a useful tool in directly treating sleep disorders.

Yoga is also a powerful tool for sleep. Yoga poses and breathing exercises can yield good results to reduce stress and anxiety, and improve sleep quality. Yoga poses are specific to each person, but some poses are better suited for relaxation and sleep.

Many yoga studios offer yoga classes for sleep which teach postures and breathing. There are also online yoga programs which can help you discover postures and incorporate them into your daily routine. Yoga postures are generally very safe and can be practiced by beginners and more advanced people alike.

Yoga and acupuncture practices can be complementary and can help you get a healthy and restorative sleep. There are also other practices such as Tai Chi and Qi Gong that can help reduce stress and relax you. Find the practice that suits you best and can help you get a restorative and healthy sleep.

Day 4: The Benefits of Herbs

When you are on your fourth day of this mini guide to beat insomnia, you can start to explore the benefits of herbs. Herbs are a natural remedy that can be used to help get back to sleep and relax the body and mind. There are many herbs that are known for their sedative and calming properties and can help you get restorative sleep.

Herbs used for treating sleep disorders can be consumed as teas or dietary supplements. The most commonly used herbs are:

- Valerian: It contains compounds that can help relax the body and soothe the mind which can help promote sleep.

- Chamomile: It is known for its anti-inflammatory and sedative properties which can help reduce agitation and help you fall asleep more easily.

- Melissa: It is often used to soothe the mind and relax before bedtime. It is also known for its antioxidant and anti-inflammatory properties.

- Passionflower: It is commonly used for its sedative and calming properties that can help to ease anxiety and promote deeper sleep.

- California Poppy: this plant contains compounds that may help reduce insomnia and help you fall asleep more easily.

- Valerian root: It is often used for its sedative and relaxing properties which can help to calm the mind and promote more restful sleep.

- Chamomile: It is known for its calming and sedative properties which can help to reduce anxiety and aid in falling asleep more easily.

- Linden Tree: It is known for its sedative and calming properties that can help relax the body and soothe the mind.

In addition to these herbs, there are other plant-based remedies that can help you get a good night's sleep. These plants include magnesium, griffonia, saffron, and melissa. The plants can be consumed in the form of tea or dietary supplements to help you get a good night's sleep.

It is very important to understand that each person responds differently to herbs. It is important to start slowly and gradually increase the dose to find the dose that best fits your condition and needs. Do not forget to consult a health professional before starting to take herbal supplements, as they may interact with other medications that you are taking.

Plants for Relaxation and Sleep

Day 4 of your mini-guide on insomnia is titled The Benefits of Herbs. Indeed, some herbs can help to get back to sleep. These herbs are both relaxing and soothing.

Among the most well-known are chamomile, escholtzia, lime tree, hawthorn, valerian, passion flower, and melissa.

Chamomile is a well-known product for its relaxing and sedative properties. Its flowers are known for its calming and stress-relieving benefits. In traditional medicine, it is used to help find sleep, to calm anxiety and to soothe anger and sadness. It can be consumed in different forms: as tea, infusion, extract or in tablet form.

California poppy (escholtzia) is a plant that is also very useful for getting back to sleep and for relaxation. It is used to fight insomnia and anxiety, and to reduce heart palpitations. It has sedative and calming properties that can help to find sleep and reduce stress. It can be consumed in the form of tea, tablets or extracts.

Linden tree is a plant that has relaxing and sedative properties. It is a very popular plant for its calming and soothing qualities. It can help to calm the nerves and relax. It can be consumed in the form of tea, infusion, tablets or extracts.

Hawthorn is a plant that is also known for its calming and sedative properties. It has been used for centuries to help relax and find sleep. It can be consumed in the form of tea, infusion, tablets or extracts.

Valerian is a plant that is known for its relaxing and sedative properties. It is used to help relax and fall asleep. It can be consumed as a tea or infusion, or in tablet or extract form.

The passion flower is a plant that is also very useful for getting back to sleep and for relaxation. It is used to fight insomnia and anxiety, and to decrease heart palpitations. It can be consumed in the form of herbal tea, tablets or extracts.

Melissa is a plant that is known for its relaxing and sedative properties. This plant is very popular for its calming and soothing virtues. It can help to calm the nerves and to relax. It can be consumed as a tea, infusion, tablets or extracts.

It is also important to note that the use of these herbs can be very useful in getting a good night's sleep and relaxing, but it is also important to consult a doctor before using them. Some herbs may interact with certain medications or other substances, and it is important to be informed and to consult a professional before doing so.

The Benefits of Herbal Teas

Herbal teas are an excellent way to regain a restorative sleep. Not only are they delicious, but they can also help fight insomnia. The plants and herbs used for herbal teas have many beneficial properties for sleep.

Herbal teas are an excellent way to provide your body with nutrients and relaxing compounds. Certain herbs are even known for their calming and hypnotic effects and can help you find sleep. The medicinal herbs that are often used for teas include:

- Chamomile: This herb is known for it's calming and sedative properties and is often used to relieve anxiety and insomnia.

- Passionflower: This plant is an excellent source of magnesium and is known for its relaxing properties.

- Melissa: This herb is known for its antispasmodic and calming properties and is often used as a natural remedy for anxiety and insomnia.

- Valerian: This herb is known for its relaxing and sedative properties and is often used to relieve insomnia and headaches.

- Peppermint: This herb is often used to relieve tension and anxiety and is also known for its sedative and relaxing properties.

- Lavender: This herb is known for its relaxing and soothing properties and is often used to help relieve anxiety and insomnia.

In addition to their relaxing and sedative properties, teas are a safe, simple and healthy way to stay hydrated and add vitamins and minerals to your diet. Teas are also rich in antioxidants that can help to counteract free radicals which can be detrimental to sleep. By drinking teas, you can enjoy the benefits of their soothing and sedative properties while staying hydrated.

Finally, one of the great advantages of herbal teas is the variety of flavors. You can add different herbs to your tea to give it a sweeter or stronger taste, depending on your preferences. Additionally, by mixing different herbs, you can get a tea that caters specifically to your needs. For example, if you want to relieve anxiety and nervousness, you can mix chamomile, peppermint and valerian.

Herbal teas are therefore an excellent solution to consider for a restorative sleep. They are easy to prepare and can help fight insomnia thanks to their relaxing and sedative properties. Finally, you can easily adapt their taste and ingredients to create the tea that suits you best.

The Benefits of Magnesium

Magnesium is an essential nutrient that can have a significant impact on your sleep quality. It helps to reduce stress and combat anxiety which are commonly at the root of insomnia. The benefits of magnesium on sleep mainly consist of:

- Reducing Stress: Magnesium is known to be calming and to relieve stress. It can help to reduce anxiety and nervous tension which are responsible for insomnia. Moreover, it is known to help improve sleep by reducing the time needed to fall asleep.

- Regulating Sleep Cycles: Magnesium can help to regulate sleep cycles by acting on the hormones that control sleep. By regulating your sleep cycle, it can help to balance your nervous system and improve your sleep quality.

- Reducing Sleep Disturbances: Magnesium can help reduce sleep disturbances such as difficulty falling asleep and staying asleep. Additionally, it can help soothe the nervous system and calm thoughts that can interfere with sleep.

- Improving Sleep Quality: Magnesium can help improve sleep quality by regulating sleep cycles and reducing the amount of time it takes to fall asleep. Additionally, by reducing stress and anxiety, it can enable deeper and better quality sleep.

In addition to its benefits for sleep, magnesium is also beneficial for your overall health. It is known to improve cardiovascular function, regulate metabolism and support the immune system. It is also beneficial for the health of bones, muscles and nerves.

Magnesium can be consumed in the form of dietary supplement or food products. Foods rich in magnesium include leafy green vegetables, nuts, seeds, cocoa, fish, meat, and legumes. Dietary supplements are also an excellent source of magnesium. It is important to read labels to ensure the product is safe and provides the right amounts of magnesium.

Day 5: Cognitive Techniques

The fifth day of your mini-guide to overcoming insomnia is dedicated to cognitive techniques. This is a set of thought and emotion management techniques designed to help insomniacs better manage and understand their anxious thoughts and negative emotions. Cognitive techniques are also useful for developing more adaptive behaviors and coping with the everyday difficulties that can cause insomnia.

Thus, for this fifth day, you are going to learn to identify negative thoughts and emotions that keep you from finding sleep and to adopt new strategies and techniques to manage them.

Advice:

- Take the time to notice and recognize what is happening in your mind and body each time you are faced with a negative thought or emotion. Be aware of how your body reacts to these thoughts and emotions and observe them without judging them.

- Learn to welcome your thoughts and emotions, even if they are negative. It is important to be aware of what is going on in your mind and to allow yourself to feel what you feel without denying or rejecting it.

- Accept and respect your boundaries. It can often be difficult to feel relaxed and calm, especially when you are under pressure or overwhelmed by negative emotions. Learn to recognize when your body and mind need time to relax and take a break.

- Develop your resilience and your ability to cope with difficult times. Resilience is a skill that can be acquired. This means that you learn to adapt to change and face the hardships of life.

- Use meditation to become aware of your mindset and your body. Meditation is a very powerful tool to become aware of what is happening inside of you. It allows you to become aware of your thoughts and emotions and to accept them without judgment.

- Learn to release your negative emotions in a constructive manner. It is important that you find healthy ways to express your negative emotions. This may include writing letters, exercising, or talking to someone.

- Learn to develop positive thoughts and focus on positives. It is important to acknowledge and thank the presence of happy moments and small positive things that happen around you. This can include thanking nature and people who are important to you.

- Learn to get rid of negative thoughts and to replace them with positive thoughts. Often, the simplest way to manage a negative thought is to replace it with a positive thought. If you find yourself thinking something negative, try to replace that thought with a more positive thought.

- Learn to control your stress and manage the stress of everyday life.

Cognitive Enhancement Techniques for Sleep Improvement

On Day 5 of your mini-guide to getting back to sleep, we are covering cognitive techniques to improve your sleep. These techniques can help to calm your mind and relax you to sleep better.

Here are some examples of cognitive techniques:

- Deep Breathing: Deep breathing can help to relax the body and calm the mind. Take your time to inhale and exhale deeply when you feel stressed or nervous.

- Positive Visualization: Positive visualization can help reduce stress and anxiety. Close your eyes and imagine a place where you feel calm and relaxed. Visualize the colors and shapes in your head and try to relax.

- Progressive Muscle Relaxation: This technique involves focusing on each muscle in your body and relaxing them one by one. This can help calm your mind and relax you.

- Positive Thinking: Try replacing negative and anxious thoughts with positive and calming ones. Replace your I can't do it with I can do it.

- Exercise: Exercise can help reduce stress and help you sleep better. Find a physical activity you enjoy and do it regularly.

- Stay active during the day: Try to stay active and occupied during the day. This can help you feel calmer and more relaxed in the evening. Try doing activities such as reading, writing, gardening, hiking, yoga, etc.

- Avoid screens: Turn off your phones, computers, and other electronic devices at least one hour before going to bed. Blue lights from screens can interfere with your sleep and prevent you from falling asleep.

- Healthy Eating: Eating healthy can help you sleep better. Avoid sugary and fatty foods before bed. Eat healthy and nutritious foods such as fruits, vegetables, whole grains, and nuts.

- Create a Comfortable Environment: Create a comfortable and calm environment in your bedroom. Make sure that your bedroom is at a comfortable temperature and that you have a comfortable mattress and pillow. You can also add items like cushions, scented candles, or soft music.

- Practice Meditation: Meditation can help to calm your mind and sleep better. Find a meditation that suits you and practice it regularly before going to bed.

Finally, cognitive techniques are a great way to manage your thoughts and sleep better. Take the time to experiment with these techniques and find the ones that work best for you. Remember that sleep is not something you can force and that cognitive techniques can help you get a restful sleep.

Cognitive Techniques for Restoring Sleep

Cognitive techniques can be an excellent way to get back to sleep and to overcome insomnia. They consist of examining the thoughts and beliefs that underlie our emotional reactions and replacing them with thoughts that are more adapted to the situation.

The main benefits of cognitive techniques are as follows:

- Reducing Stress and Anxiety: Cognitive techniques can help you identify and modify thoughts and beliefs that increase your level of stress and anxiety.

- Increase Sense of Control: Cognitive Techniques Help You Better Understand and Manage Stressful Circumstances That Are the Source of Your Insomnia.

- Improving Sleep Quality: Once you have identified and changed the thoughts that cause insomnia, you can start to sleep better and feel more rested.

- Reducing Sleep Disorders: Cognitive techniques can help reduce many forms of sleep disorders, including insomnia, nightmares, sleep apnea, etc.

- Emotion Management: Cognitive techniques can help you develop strategies to better manage your emotions and increase your ability to relax and sleep better.

- Improving Quality of Life: Cognitive techniques can help you better manage stress and anxiety, which are often the cause of insomnia and improve the quality of your life.

To use cognitive techniques to overcome insomnia, the first step is to start by examining the thoughts and beliefs that are at the root of your insomnia. You can use tools such as journaling to identify the thoughts and beliefs that are at the root of your insomnia. Once you have identified these thoughts and beliefs, you can begin to replace them with more appropriate thoughts for the situation.

The second step is to set up strategies to manage stress and anxiety which are often the root causes of insomnia. You can use relaxation techniques such as meditation, yoga, breathing exercises, etc. to help reduce the stress and anxiety that may be preventing you from sleeping.

The third step is to modify your environment to promote sleep. This can include things like maintaining a comfortable bedroom temperature, setting up a relaxing bedtime ritual, staying away from screens and noise, etc.

Finally, the fourth step is to be more active and adopt healthy sleep habits such as physical exercise, healthy eating and regular sleep schedules. These habits can help to improve the quality and duration of your sleep.

By following these four steps, you can learn to use cognitive techniques to regain sleep and conquer insomnia. The key is to make sure you take the time to understand your thoughts and beliefs and use strategies.

Cognitive Techniques for Preventing Insomnia

Day 5 is dedicated to cognitive techniques to prevent insomnia. These techniques aim to modify the thoughts and behaviors that maintain insomnia and to provide better management and understanding of the factors that influence sleep.

During insomnia, it is common for thoughts to accumulate and cause anxiety and restlessness that prevent sleep. Cognitive techniques allow working with these thoughts and being aware of them in order to replace them with more positive and calming thoughts.

A good practice is to take the time to sit down and write down the thoughts and beliefs that are preventing us from falling asleep. Once these thoughts are identified, the following are cognitive techniques that can be used to replace them with more positive and calming thoughts:

- Questioning or Challenging Thoughts: This involves challenging negative automatic thoughts by putting yourself in someone else's shoes and objectively asking if these thoughts are really justified.

- Debunking Thoughts and Beliefs: It is about recognizing that some thoughts and beliefs are so deeply ingrained that they have become realities for us. Therefore, it is important to question and confront them in order to reduce their influence on our thoughts and sleep.

- Practicing Acceptance and Tolerance: It is important to recognize the feelings and thoughts that are hard to accept and to accept them as part of oneself. This allows for a distance to be taken from the thoughts and to look at them objectively.

- Muscle Relaxation: These exercises involve contracting and relaxing muscles to help relax the body and quiet the mind.

- Visualization: It is to use one's imagination to visualize oneself in a state of relaxation, which can help to create a calmer and more tranquil mental state.

- Deep and Controlled Breathing: Taking the time to breathe deeply and calmly can help reduce stress and relieve muscle tension.

- Meditation and Relaxation: Meditation and relaxation are powerful tools to help center and release mentally and physically.

- Planning and Proactive Management: It is important to take steps to manage and reduce factors that contribute to difficulty sleeping, such as reducing caffeine and alcohol consumption and avoiding naps during the day.

Finally, another effective method is to replace negative thoughts with positive and beneficial thoughts. This can be done by focusing on positive things and committing to find ways to cope with difficulties.

In summary, cognitive techniques can help prevent insomnia by altering the thoughts and behaviors that maintain insomnia and by providing better management and understanding of the factors that influence sleep.

Day 6: Screening for Insomnia-Related Diseases

On the sixth day of our mini guide, we will talk about diseases related to insomnia and what you should be aware of.

It is really essential to remember that you should always consult your doctor if you think your sleep is affected by an illness. Sleep disorders can be caused by a variety of illnesses, including:

- Parkinson's Disease: a neurological disease which causes trembling and slow movements. People with Parkinson's Disease often have difficulty getting restorative sleep and waking up early in the morning.

- Respiratory Insufficiency: This occurs when the body does not receive enough oxygen to function properly. People with respiratory insufficiency may suffer from insomnia, daytime drowsiness, and poor sleep quality.

- High Blood Pressure: High blood pressure can lead to difficulty sleeping, frequent nighttime awakenings, and poor sleep quality.

- Anxiety and Depression Disorders: Anxiety and depression disorders can lead to difficulty falling asleep and staying asleep. People suffering from these disorders can also experience nighttime awakenings and poor sleep quality.

- Restless Leg Syndrome: This syndrome causes discomfort and unpleasant sensations in the legs that can disturb sleep.

- Movement Disorders: Movement disorders can cause involuntary body movements that can disrupt sleep quality.

- Thyroid disorders: an underactive thyroid can cause difficulty falling asleep and staying asleep, as well as poor quality sleep.

- Bladder Disease: People suffering from this disease may experience frequent urges to urinate, which can affect sleep.

- Sleep Apnea Syndrome: Sleep Apnea Syndrome is characterized by repeated pauses in breathing during sleep. People with Sleep Apnea Syndrome may wake up multiple times in the night and have difficulty returning to restorative sleep.

It is important to consult a doctor for any persistent sleep disorder. Your doctor can diagnose and treat any underlying illnesses that could be causing your insomnia. They can also help you find ways to manage and ease your sleep.

Insomnia-Related Diseases

Diseases related to insomnia can be as varied as the symptoms that can be observed. Chronic insomnia or night awakenings can be a sign of a psychological problem, hormonal imbalance or a more serious medical condition.

- Mental Health Disorders: Mental health disorders are among the most common causes of sleep disturbances. People suffering from disorders such as anxiety, depression, and eating disorders are more likely to suffer from insomnia. Anxiety and depression can lead to persistent insomnia and treatment of these disorders can help to relieve insomnia.

- Movement and Sleep Disorders: Movement and sleep disorders, such as narcolepsy, can cause nighttime awakenings and difficulty falling asleep. Narcolepsy is a neurological disorder characterized by periods of excessive sleepiness and a tendency to fall asleep in inappropriate situations. Other symptoms of narcolepsy include hallucinations and an inability to stay awake for extended periods of time. Other movement and sleep disorders, such as restless leg syndrome, can also lead to sleep disruption.

- Hormonal Imbalance: Sleep disturbances can also be a sign of hormonal imbalance. Women are more likely to suffer from insomnia during their menstrual and menopausal periods. Thyroid and melatonin disorders can also lead to sleep disturbances.

- Circadian Rhythm Disorders: Circadian rhythm disorders are a common cause of insomnia. These disorders are characterized by disturbances of the natural rhythm of sleep and wake cycles. Circadian rhythm disorders may be related to night shift work, time changes, or jet lag. People suffering from these disorders may have difficulty falling asleep and staying asleep for prolonged periods of time.

- Allergies and Respiratory Conditions: Allergies and respiratory conditions can also be the cause of difficulty sleeping and nighttime awakenings. Allergic people can suffer from nasal congestion and an allergic cough that can disturb their sleep. Respiratory conditions such as asthma can also lead to sleep disruption.

- Cardiovascular and neurological conditions: Cardiovascular and neurological conditions can also be the cause of sleep disturbances. Cardiovascular disorders can lead to a feeling of chest tightness and persistent insomnia. Neurological disorders, such as multiple sclerosis, can also result in regular nocturnal awakenings.

- Drug and Alcohol Use: Excessive use of drugs and alcohol can lead to sleep disturbances. Alcohol can disrupt sleep and cause night awakenings.

Medications for Treating Insomnia

It is clear that medications can be an effective means for treating insomnia. However, they are only recommended as a last resort. The most commonly prescribed medications for insomnia are hypnotics, which are sleeping pills. They are usually prescribed for moderate to severe symptoms and should only be used for a limited period of time to avoid side effects and the risk of addiction.

Hypnotics can be sedatives, which are lighter and have fewer side effects. They can also be hypnotic analgesics, which are stronger and have more side effects. Doctors can also prescribe antidepressants to help reduce insomnia. Antidepressants can help reduce anxiety and regulate the wake-sleep cycle.

Before taking medication to treat insomnia, it is important to understand the potential side effects and risks. The most common side effects of sleeping pills are drowsiness, headaches, grogginess, and confusion. They can also lead to memory problems, fainting, dizziness, and mood swings. It is important to discuss with your doctor all side effects and the possibility of dependence before taking medication for insomnia.

Medication may be an effective solution for treating insomnia, but it is important to take the time to consult with a health professional to determine the best solution for you. Your doctor can help you to determine which medication and what dose you should take.

The benefits of medications for treating insomnia include:

- Almost immediate improvement of insomnia state.

- They can help to restore sleep cycles more quickly.

- They can also relieve stress and anxiety which can cause insomnia.

However, there are also drawbacks to taking medications to treat insomnia, including:

- Possible side effects such as headaches, dizziness, drowsiness, confusion, or deep sleep.

- Physical or psychological dependency.

- Medications take time to work and are not a long-term solution for treating insomnia.

Before taking medications to treat insomnia, it is important to understand potential side effects and risks. It is also important to talk to your doctor to make sure that the prescribed medications are right for your needs and your health. It is also important to follow the doctor's instructions and never take medications without talking to your doctor first.

Alternative Methods

Alternative methods for treating and preventing insomnia are an excellent option for those who do not have the time or money to visit a healthcare professional. There are a variety of treatments available, including:

- Meditation and relaxation. Meditation and relaxation are powerful tools that can help to calm the body and mind and relieve stress. Meditation and relaxation exercises can help you relax, concentrate, and better manage levels of stress that can contribute to insomnia.

- Cognitive-Behavioral Therapy. Cognitive-behavioral therapy (CBT) is a psychological approach that aims to modify behaviors or thoughts that can contribute to insomnia. Tools such as sleep journaling, cognitive restructuring, and behavior therapy can help treat and prevent insomnia.

- Herbal supplements. Herbal supplements such as melatonin, valerian, magnesium and tryptophan may help improve the quality and duration of sleep. However, before taking herbal supplements, it is recommended to consult a doctor or qualified healthcare professional to discuss potential risks and benefits.

- Physical exercise. In addition to being a great way to have fun, exercise can help to relieve stress and improve the quality and duration of sleep. Regular exercise can also help to reduce the symptoms of insomnia.

- Dietary modifications. Changing dietary habits can help to improve the quality and length of sleep. A healthy and balanced diet can help to reduce the symptoms of insomnia, while avoiding foods and drinks that are stimulating before bedtime can also help to improve sleep.

- Acupuncture. Acupuncture is a medical practice that can help to relieve stress and improve the quality and duration of sleep. The specific points that are stimulated can help to reduce the symptoms of insomnia.

- Sunlight. Adequate exposure to sunlight can help to trigger sleep hormones and improve the quality and length of sleep. Ultraviolet light can also help to regulate the wake-sleep cycle and resolve insomnia symptoms.

- Yoga and Tai Chi. Yoga and Tai Chi are forms of meditation that can help to calm the body and mind and improve the quality and duration of sleep. Yoga and Tai Chi exercises can help to reduce the symptoms of insomnia and better manage stress and anxiety.

- Complementary methods. Many complementary methods can help to relieve stress and improve the quality and length of sleep. Massages, baths, yoga, meditation and relaxation techniques may all be of help.

Day 7: When to See a Doctor?

At the ultimate stage, when all other attempts to regain normal sleep have failed, it may be time to consult a doctor. A doctor can assess the underlying causes of your insomnia and advise on possible treatments.

First of all, prepare for your medical appointment by taking note of the symptoms you have experienced and reflecting on the questions you want to ask. This will give your doctor a better picture of your condition and overall health.

Your doctor may ask you questions about your lifestyle and the circumstances that occurred before and during your attempt to sleep. He or she may ask you to fill out a physical and psychological assessment questionnaire, and may also perform blood tests and physical examinations to evaluate your overall health.

There are several optional treatments available for treating insomnia, including medications, relaxation practices, behavior modifications, and therapy. Medications are often used to treat short-term insomnia but may not be beneficial in the long run. Relaxation techniques and behavior modifications are long-term strategies to get to sleep and stay asleep throughout the night. It is also possible that your doctor may recommend that you seek the advice of a psychologist to help manage your stress and worries which may interfere with your sleep.

No matter what treatment your doctor suggests, it is important to remember that every person is different and what works for one may not necessarily work for the other. If your doctor prescribes a treatment, make sure to follow the instructions and contact your doctor if you notice any changes in your sleep or any unwanted side effects.

In addition to medications, your doctor may also recommend lifestyle modifications to help you get back to normal sleep. For example, the doctor may advise you to make changes to your diet and lifestyle, reduce consumption of stimulants such as caffeine and alcohol, and adopt rituals to help you fall asleep and stay asleep.

It is important to remember that excessive use of sleep medications is not safe and can worsen your insomnia. If you are taking sleep medications, make sure to take them at recommended doses and only for a short period of time. Do not take any other sleep medications without your doctor's permission.

Finally, once treatment has begun, carefully monitor your progress and consult your doctor if you notice any changes or if you are not getting the results you expected. With the right tools and information, you can learn to manage your diabetes.

When insomnia becomes chronic

When insomnia becomes chronic, it is time to consult a doctor. Certain factors can be the cause of these nighttime awakenings. That is why, it is important to recognize the signs and symptoms of chronic insomnia and to consult a doctor for a diagnosis and an appropriate treatment.

The causes of chronic insomnia can be multiple:

- Chronic pain or pain related to an illness or injury.

- Stress and anxiety which can be related to mental health or everyday life events.

- An uncomfortable or noisy sleeping environment.

- Hormonal changes related to menopause, pregnancy, or medication use.

- Imbalance of thyroid hormones, nutritional deficiencies, or metabolic diseases.

- The Side Effects of Medications.

- Unhealthy sleep habits and poor sleep hygiene.

If you notice that your insomnia is not improving despite lifestyle changes, relaxation sessions, and natural remedies, it is time to consult a doctor. Your doctor can prescribe medications to help relieve symptoms and help you treat the underlying cause. Your doctor can also refer you to a qualified health professional who can recommend therapies and advice to help you better manage your problem.

It is also important to try to understand why insomnia has become chronic and reduce or eliminate the factors that may be causing it. Sleep environment can be a major factor, as well as stress and anxiety. Try to find ways to manage your stress and worries, such as relaxing and practicing meditation exercises before bed.

You can also try natural remedies such as medicinal plants, aromatherapy, essential oils, and herbs to help ease your symptoms and improve your sleep quality. These remedies can be very beneficial for some people, but it is important to consult your doctor before beginning to use them.

Finally, it's important to recognize that chronic insomnia can be a sign of an underlying disorder, such as an anxiety or depressive disorder or a medical illness. In this case, your doctor may direct you to a qualified health professional who can help you identify the underlying cause and develop a treatment plan tailored to your needs.

The Medical Consequences of Insomnia

The medical consequences related to insomnia can be very serious and they are numerous. Poor quality of sleep has impacts on the body and can cause health problems such as:

- Difficulties concentrating and remembering

- A general decrease in energy

- Increased Risk of Accidents

- Depression

- Weight Gain

- An increase in the risks of heart disease, type 2 diabetes and respiratory illnesses

- Increase in Stress

- A Decrease in Immune Defenses

Furthermore, insomnia can have an impact on the quality of life in general. It can affect the ability to work and even function normally in society. People suffering from insomnia are more likely to experience chronic fatigue and mood swings, which can affect their relationships with their loved ones and colleagues.

Finally, and most importantly, quality sleep is essential for good psychological and physical functioning. The negative effects on health caused by insomnia are numerous and can be very serious. That is why it is essential to take measures to treat insomnia and regain good sleep. If your attempts to resolve your insomnia have failed, it is important to consult a doctor to find adequate solutions.

When to See a Doctor for Insomnia

Sleep is vital for health and the proper functioning of the body, which is why it is essential to get medical treatment for insomnia. However, before consulting a doctor for your insomnia, it is important to understand how this illness manifests itself.

Doctors are generally able to diagnose a sleep disorder based on the patient's symptoms and medical history. Furthermore, they can also advise you on ways to improve your sleep.

When consulting a doctor about your insomnia, it is important to provide detailed information about your symptoms and sleeping habits. Here are some key elements to mention:

- When did you start suffering from insomnia?

- What are your symptoms?

- Do you wake up at night or are you unable to fall asleep?

- What is your medical history?

- Do you have healthy sleeping habits?

- Do you take any medication or supplements?

- It is also important to mention if you suffer from any associated disorders: anxiety, depression, stress, etc. This information will help the doctor better assess your condition and provide you with the appropriate treatment.

Finally, it is advisable to discuss your expectations and goals with your doctor. For example, do you just want to improve the quality of your sleep or be able to fall asleep more easily? The doctor can then tailor the treatment to your specific needs.

www.ingramcontent.com/pod-product-compliance
Lightning Source LLC
Chambersburg PA
CBHW071106260726
48661CB00006B/2484